Stop Your Nail Biting!
Permanently

See real pictures and cases at:
http://www.stopyournailbiting.com

Gilbreth Brown

Stop Your Nail Biting!

Reader's Rave:

I received the book a few days ago, read it in its entirety, and started the technique right away. I just have to say THANK YOU Mr. Brown!!! It is nothing short of a miracle. It not just the technique itself, but the background information that is written about the habit that is so valuable. I have not bitten my nails even once in three days. That seems like a short time, but for me it is a record. I can't believe it was so simple and yet so effective. After I read the book I was a little mad because I thought, "I actually paid for a book to tell me this?!" But then I started it, it worked immediately, and now I think that is a very small price to pay for such freedom!

I have been a 24 year sufferer of this habit (I am 30 right now) and my nails have been bitten down as far as they will go. They were so short that I had to start a new habit: peeling the layers of my nails until my nailbed bled. I have had many complications such as getting nail pieces stuck in my teeth, in my gums, and in my throat. I have also had infections on my fingers and in my gums. Also, since I am a scientist, nail biting is not just a bad habit - it can be highly dangerous what with all the chemicals that I work with. I was all but hopeless, having tried everything from bad tasting hot pepper polish, bitter cremes, weekly manicures, acrylic nails, and bandaging my fingers. The only time that my nails grew was when I was ten years old and I could not reach my fingers because my arm was in a cast; they lasted a matter of hours before they were torn and chewed off.

This post may be premature, but I am confident that I will be able to keep this up, knowing what I know now. I will send the before and after digital pictures in a few months. I can't wait to see my long, long nails!

If you are having doubts about buying this book and you are trying to get more information from reading posts on this forum, all I can say is, "just by the book!!" In my opinion, the background (i.e., the secondary habit) is more important than the technique itself, so just knowing the technique will probably not help you anyway.

Just one more note: I was not even that motivated to stop my nail biting habit. I just thought that I "should", so I bought the book. The knowledge and the technique that Mr. Brown provides is THAT powerful.

More Readers Rave:

This is confirmation that I have received the package. I have spent the weekend reading the material, and I can say that when I finished reading the solution chapter I was actually laughing... Laughing because for 25 years I have felt powerless to stop this habit - and yet in one page you describe a technique that I know will work. I just had to laugh! So now, after three days I have still only applied the method a few times - the strength seems to come from knowing a way out!

We received your book this past week and I started the technique right away. I'm on day six of no nail biting and it's been so much easier than I ever would have thought. Truly can't believe it's been six days already! I can't wait to show the family at Christmas that after probably close to 30 years of nail biting, I have finally kicked the habit!

Hi Gil, thanks very much for enquiring. I have read the book and not bitten my nails since. I am scared I will go back to the habit as I have been doing it for so long. It has been about five weeks since I started and my nails are not fully grown yet but they are a vast improvement. I hear they take about 6 months to look good after biting them for so long. My husband is amazed, I have been trying to stop for years (I am 31 and a mother to 6 great kids) and each time he has encouraged me and tried to help me. Each time I have gone back to the habit about four to six weeks later and I felt I had not only let myself down but let him down too. The only time I haven't bitten my nails for a long time is when I have just had a baby (maybe there is something behind that!).

When I see people in shops and bars and restaurants who bite their nails and are complete strangers (none of my friends have this terrible habit) I feel like giving them your website to help them. But I think it might be a bit rude! As you say in your book it is a real burden and one feels quite embarrassed about doing such a childish thing when one is a grown up. Thank you so, so much for sharing your technique and I will promote your website when I can.

Stop Your Nail Biting
1st Edition, 2004
©Stopyournailbiting.com
245/2 Sukhumvit Soi 21 (asoke)
Klongtoey, Wattana
Bangkok Thailand 10110
A special thank you goes to Barbara Ardinger,
whose editing and input was excellent and highly welcomed.
Design and typesetting, Roy Diment, VRG.
www.members.shaw.ca/vrg
Cover, Roy Diment
Printed in Canada.

Note To Librarians: A cataloguing record for this book that includes the U.S. Library of Congress Classification number, the Library of Congress Call number and the Dewey Decimal cataloguing code is available from the National Library of Canada. The complete cataloguing record can be obtained from the National Library's online database at: www.nlc-bnc.ca/amicus/index-e.html

ISBN 1-4120-2364-5

TRAFFORD

This book was published *on-demand* in cooperation with Trafford Publishing. On-demand publishing is a unique process and service of making a book available for retail sale to the public taking advantage of on-demand manufacturing and Internet marketing. **On-demand publishing** includes promotions, retail sales, manufacturing, order fulfilment, accounting and collecting royalties on behalf of the author.

Suite 6E, 2333 Government St., Victoria, B.C. V8T 4P4, CANADA
Phone   250-383-6864   Toll-free   1-888-232-4444 (Canada & US)
Fax   250-383-6804   E-mail   sales@trafford.com
Web site www.trafford.com   TRAFFORD PUBLISHING IS A DIVISION OF TRAFFORD HOLDINGS, LTD.
Trafford Catalogue # 04-0192   www.trafford.com/robots/04-0192.html

10   9   8   7   6

Stop Your Nail Biting!
Permanently

Gilbreth Brown
Trafford Publishing
2004

ABOUT THE AUTHOR

Gilbreth Brown has been living in Asia for approximately the last ten years. He is originally from Providence, Rhode Island. Born on February 8, 1966 he grew up in Providence before relocating with his parents and siblings to western RI. Currently, he is residing in Bangkok Thailand. Although he is a frequent guest speaker and contributor to leading business publications, this is his first book.

Gilbreth is an avid reader, and most often you will find him browsing the self-help section of the neighbourhood bookstore. His personal quest to better himself led him on a long search for the cure to his nail biting problem. The results of that search are contained here.

Gilbreth Brown holds a Bachelors of Science from Boston University, a Masters in Japanese Business Studies from Chaminade University of Honolulu, and an MBA from Columbia Business School. As a result of a long stay in Asia, he is highly proficient in both Japanese and the Thai language.

He welcomes comments at any time at
http://www.stopyournailbiting.com

For Gator and Q, two stray dogs that have recently come into and brightened my life in so many ways. I could only wish to have a portion of their courage and beauty. Now if they would only leave the kitchen cabinets alone…

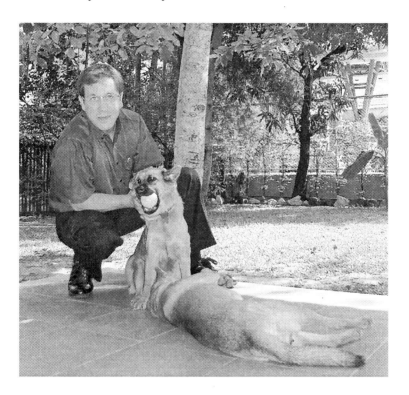

Contents

1

FOREWORD

As a habitual, but now cured, nail biter for many years of my life, I understand this problem. I feel great compassion for other sufferers. If you are currently a nail biter, I share your frustration and grief. I am here to work with you to truly and permanently rid yourself of this frustrating habit.

Having bitten and chewed my fingers from roughly six years of age until my early thirties, I never thought that I would be sitting down to write a book about how to permanently cure this strange habit. I am thirty-seven now, and I have not bitten my nails since I found and refined the cure for this bad habit many years ago. The secret is given in this book. After you have completed the reading, I am highly confident that you, too, will succeed in never biting your nails again.

I have worked with countless people helping them to overcome this bad habit and find freedom from their despair. Contained in these pages is a technique that some of the people I have helped call *nothing short of a miracle*. I am pleased to receive letters, e-mails, and phone calls from people who continue to thank me years after they successfully used the technique contained in these pages.

I have many reasons for writing this book. First, I want to empower the world's habitual nail biters by providing them with knowledge of their habit. Knowledge is power. It will provide the foundation to our ultimate success at overcoming the habit.

Second, there is little contemporary data available related to adult nail biting. The data that I have found is dated, and often buried in obscure medical and psychiatric journals. I want to brush off the dust and bring this habit into the open so that habitual nail biters can receive the help that they deserve.

Third, I also want to bring into the mainstream a documented but little known cure to this habit. My aim is to spread the word that problem nail biting can be solved. If you are a habitual nail biter and you are suffering in silence, my goal is to help you with a cure that I believe is close to perfect. After you have finished reading this book, you will see that you can finally and permanently rid yourself of this unsightly habit.

I believe that there are two reasons that reformed nail-biters are so elated once they have successfully quit the habit. The first reason is obvious—their fingertips are attractive! They enjoy eating in public more, shaking hands more often, and exchanging business cards openly. Reformed nail-biters enjoy going to the manicurist. They are unafraid of showing their hands in public. For non-biters, the significance of this statement is difficult to comprehend. I tell my own story a little later on. You will understand how I came to dread exchanging business cards because people would look at my hands with pity or disgust.

Secondly, and perhaps more importantly, ridding oneself of this awful habit has an immediate and significant positive impact on a person's sense of self-worth. This burst of positive energy releases the habitual biter from a variety of accompanying other insecurities or related baggage. It is as if someone has pushed away a thin veil that hovers over or around a nail biter's psyche or mental state. Once the veil is gone, confidence and emotional well being improve significantly. For me, my happiness at being cured spilled over into other areas of my life. I gained higher self confidence and a feeling that I could now surmount any of life's hurdles. In essence, I was no longer a prisoner of the habit. I gained an incredible feeling of freedom.

I will go into more detail in the following pages, but for the moment, please know that I frequently receive calls and mail from many people who say that I have changed their life for the better and in a heretofore unimagined way.

As a reformed nail biter, I understand how personal this habit can be. Wherever possible, I have included in the text you are about to read an account of my own battle with this habit. You will come to understand that you are not alone in the world. In our case, misery definitely welcomes company!

I am here with you, accompanying you on your journey to finally and permanently divorce you from this mind bogglingly difficult-to-break habit. You will be most successful in your quest if you read this book closely and in its entirety. You may be tempted to jump ahead to the solution chapter. *Don't do it!*

By reading and understanding the background of nail biting, you are forming a solid intellectual foundation upon which you can now confidently stand. You will be able to attack the habit with both knowledge and a powerful cure. The combination is a serious and very well documented therapeutic approach.

See my web site—http://www.stopyournailbiting.com—for success stories and pictures.

Before I set you off on this journey though, what I require from you is a commitment. You alone hold the keys to your success. You will learn to be responsible for your own behavior and for banishing this habit forever from your life. I am confident that, like countless other folks who have used the technique I am about to describe, you will find freedom.

Before we begin, I would like to recount an experience that I had during my very first day of graduate school in New York. Typically, new students gather in a large auditorium at the start of the semester. One by one, they stand up and try to introduce themselves to their classmates in a novel way that will impress their peers and set their social stage for the duration of school.

As the self-introductions went around the room I struggled to find something interesting and witty to say that would grab the attention from a room full of extremely bright and motivated business students. At the time, I had been free of the nail biting habit for about six months. I was proud of myself and eager to share my healing experience. I hoped that I could help other people. But I was not prepared for what happened next.

As my turn came, I stood up, and briefly mentioned that I had just broken my nail biting habit and that anyone else wishing to do so could come to me for help. The room immediately went silent. I stood there beaming, waiting for applause, naïvely thinking that my fellow students would share my happiness. To my horror, everyone broke into raucous laughter. Red faced and highly embarrassed, I shrank back into my seat. *Great way to start graduate school*, I said to myself, envisioning lunch alone for the next two years with everyone snickering behind my back.

That afternoon, however, and over the next few days, I was privately approached by 20 or 25 students. Each one secretly confided in me that they bit their nails and wished to stop—at almost any cost. This was my first foray into helping people vanquish this bad habit. Graduate school turned into the laboratory in which I was able to refine the technique presented in these pages. I will never forget that day I stood up. I will never regret making a monkey out of myself. Because of that memorable day, I am now able to share the secret of success with you.

Good luck in all your journeys and please keep in touch by logging into my web site and sharing your experience with our community. Read on now. Learn how you can finally and permanently cure yourself of nail biting.

2

NAIL BITING DEFINED

Most people are familiar with nail biting, but few people truly *understand* the habit. While nail biting is a habit that most people suffer from at least some time in their life, it is something we rarely discuss. Often, we are simply too embarrassed.

Children who bite their nails are scolded by their parents and told to *stop it*, or to *grow up*. Alternatively, adults who bite their nails are deemed to be *anxious* or *nervous*. Few people who witness a nail biter sawing away can offer aid in any form. More often, they pity, criticize, or chastise the biter. We try to avoid discussing the topic at all for fear of embarrassing the biter or ourselves. Misunderstanding reigns. Because of their acute embarrassment and lack of understanding of the habit, nail-biters themselves rarely raise the issue. Often, there is no place to turn for help.

What results is that nail biting tends to be an extremely personal habit that forces the habitual biter to suffer in private. Unlike Alcoholics Anonymous, overeating seminars, anger-management groups, or other group-based therapies, there are few nail biting support groups. To the best of my knowledge, there are no classes to attend, no community support groups, no textbooks, and no doctors that specialize in therapy for habitual nail-biters. Although some psychiatrists or psychotherapists might offer hypnotherapy or similar treatment, most would probably admit that they were flying in the dark. Given the prevalence of the habit, I find this lack of treatment help puzzling.

Before continuing into a detailed description of nail biting, I will pause and clarify terminology. Throughout the text you are about to read, I refer to nail biting as a bad *habit*. This is correct I believe, as most dictionaries define the term *nail biting* as a *nervous habit*. However, it is my personal opinion that it is not inappropriate to use stronger terminology to describe the behavior. This might include phrases like *condition, ailment, affliction,* or *malady.* In the past, I could easily have used these terms to describe my own habit. I want more importance placed on the problem.

However, I recognize that nail biting may not meet the generally accepted clinical criteria for these more serious sounding classifications. Although nail-biters may think of themselves as afflicted, it is important to understand that nail biting is frequently merely an odd behavior. It is highly habituated behavior, but nevertheless behavior that can be changed. It is a bad habit, and very often nothing more serious than that.

A TWO-STEP PROCESS:

Let us begin by breaking the behavior down into two separate processes. The nail biting habit is unique in this regard, and I urge you to pause here for some serious reflection. You should fully understand this material, for it is critical to the success of the treatment. To be fully and permanently cured, you must understand and recognize your own behavior by internalizing the material I am about to share with you. Spend time on this section.

Although it seems counter-intuitive to do so, I will start by defining Step 2 of the two-step process that makes up the overall nail biting habit. Then I will complete the definition by shedding light on a set of well recognized behaviours that almost always precede nail biting. I will refer to these two steps of the habit as the primary and secondary habits.

Step 2 (the primary habit) defined

Nail biting is the habit of periodically and habitually biting, picking, tearing, ripping, gnawing, gouging, licking, smoothing, pruning, or performing any other self-inflicted action targeted toward mutilating the ends of one's fingers. (I will address toenail and cheek biting and other forms of self-pruning later in the book.) This pruning is performed lightly or heavily. It can result in pain and bloodletting. It is not necessarily confined to a single hand or specific fingers, but can include both hands and any or all fingers.

Incidentally, *nail biting is frequently not just about the nail.* Often, the skin around the nail, including the cuticle, is equally appealing to the biter. The entire fingertip is often the target of drawn out attacks in which whole areas of skin around the nails are picked or peeled away.

The result of primary nail biting or self-pruning is a set of fingernails that are heavily cropped. The surrounding skin is deeply gouged, reddened, bloody, or cosmetically irregular in appearance. Pain, swelling, and bleeding are not uncommon. Typically, nail biters also have a peculiar behavior in which whole piles of tiny bits of flesh and nail accumulate on the table or, unknowingly, in the folds of the shirt they are wearing at the time of their self-dismemberment. I have often seen what looks like snow falling from the shirt of a serious nail biter as they rise to their feet.

A Personal Side Note

From approximately the age of six, I was a habitual and extremely devoted nail biter. In my case, nail biting *is not the best word for my habit. I did not actually* bite. *Instead, I would pick and tear the skin around the nails until there was simply nothing left. Often, blood would run. I dismembered my fingernails, and then moved to the skin around my cropped nails. Each finger was a systematically attacked, and there was little pattern to my behavior. I was frequently distressed with the condition of my hands.*

For more than 25 years, I tried desperately to stop. In good times, a week would pass without engaging in this awful habit. Soon after however, I could undo a week's worth of growth in one short session watching TV or sitting in a taxi. I would arrive back from where I had started—with painful, unsightly fingertips. The cycle was cruel, and it bore heavily down upon my psyche. I simply could not understand why I did not have the will power to control my own behavior! What was wrong with me?

CRITICAL MATERIAL!

Step 1 (the secondary habit) defined

Read carefully, for what I will tell you here is *important to the cure.*

For our purposes, nail biting as a defined end-to-end behavior also includes the secondary habit or act of systematically *inspecting* the nails in minute detail in search of any irregularity in the skin or nail. Once located, the irregularity becomes the focal point of attention. Biters cannot help themselves, and typically obsesses over small defects in the nail or skin. They start biting and tearing. The defect provides the excuse needed to justify the behavior. *If I can only clean this little ugly bit off...* is how the thinking transpires.

This secondary habit of *careful inspection* almost always precedes the actual or primary habit of nail biting. Watch yourself carefully. Learn to recognize the moments when you discretely and subtlety draw up your hands and turn them this way and that looking for an entry into the actual picking. You are searching for a small gouge, a hangnail, a bit of irregular skin, or any kind of deformed area. Often, you are not even aware of either primary or secondary habit behavior.

To emphasize this important point, let me repeat it. Typically, habitual nail biters carefully inspect and feel around the ends of their fingers. They are searching for titbits to focus on *just before* engaging in their primary nail biting behavior. As soon as they find a piece of skin or nail that is slightly irregular or out of place, they target the offending bit of flesh or nail with vicious attention in an attempt to smooth it out or clean it away.

This secondary searching habit is the typical start to a ten or fifteen minute session of primary nail picking and or biting. Once located, a small hangnail preoccupies the habit owner's mind. No amount of will power or mental strength can overcome the desire to clear it off or pick it away.

Often, the person in question is not even aware of their behavior, either during the secondary search or during primary biting occurrences. Both the searching behavior and the primary nail biting can be entirely unconscious, and I have witnessed nail biters openly performing ritualistic *search and destroy* missions even as I talk to them about their own behavior!

Because nail-biters often bite unconsciously, friends or family often try to reach out and grab the hand of the biter in a futile attempt to force him or her to cease and desist. Suddenly aware, the biter stops; but only for the moment, and usually only out of embarrassment. In almost all cases, such measures by friends and family are only temporarily effective. The nail biter simply invents better ways to hide the habit.

With few exceptions, almost every one of the persons that I have worked with has told me that, yes; indeed, they often bite their nails or prune their fingertips *after* a casual glance down at their fingers or after a *feeling session* (gliding one finger down the length of another, feeling for pits or gouges).

During these sessions, subjects are looking for a small irregularity on which to blame their pruning. Many have told me about an overwhelming desire or urge to smooth out the edges of their nails or fingertips.

As one person told me,
I would feel lightly along each of my fingers until I found a small bump or a hangnail. This would provide an almost frustratingly pleasurable feeling of satisfaction. Once having located a target, I had the excuse that I needed to start peeling and smoothing away. However, the behavior is a vicious cycle. The more you smooth, the more irregular your fingers become, and the maddening cycle starts all over again. You end up adding fuel to your own fire. (Cindy, Housewife)

To summarize, nail biting includes two self-destructive behaviors that together form the habit. First, the absent-minded search or inspection (secondary habit) happens. This I refer to as *targeting*. Second, the actual nail biting (primary habit) occurs following the targeting. Together, these two behaviors form the overall nail biting habit.

For you to permanently eradicate the habit, you must recognize both primary and secondary behaviors as integral parts of the total habit. You must also learn to recognize the times when you are engaging in unconscious primary or secondary behavior. To do so, we will set up an alarm in your mind that will allow you to shift recognition of these behaviors into your consciousness. Later in this book, I will give you a powerful technique for how to do this.

It is important to recognize and understand both primary and secondary behaviors. If targeting can be eliminated, we are well on our way to eradicating the habit at its roots – permanently, and effectively. Other methods of nail biting habit control cannot treat the habit at its inception. As a cure for nail biting, I believe that the technique I will describe to you is far superior to any other in the world.

3

A COMMON HABIT

While conducting research for this book, I discovered that there are few sources of information with regard to how many people in the world bite or pick their nails. The data that does exist is highly fragmented, widely varied, and occasionally contradictory. About the only thing that experts can agree on is that there are *a lot* of people in the world who suffer from the habit.

The important message here is that *you are not alone*. Once I came to this realization myself, I felt comforted to know that I was not alone in my suffering. It is like the feeling I had as a child on sleepless nights. Listening through the window to the noises of the surrounding city was somehow comforting. These sounds told me that I was not the only one awake at the time. The same can be said of nail biting. *You are not alone*.

There are many people in the world who share this habit, people from all walks of life, societies, demographics, cultures, and ages. Your habit may be personal, but that does not mean you have a monopoly on the behavior.

Regarding the exact number of people who bite their nails, only a handful of reliable studies are available. Good contemporary data is even more difficult to locate. It could be that the habit is not considered serious or important enough to attract clinical research funding. I imagine that the world's nail biters would differ in opinion!

The best estimate I have seen is that somewhere from *20% to 30% of the general population has this habit* at any one time (Ballinger 1970). Ballinger found that, according to age, the prevalence of nail biting ranges from 18.4% (up to nine years) to as high as 35.2 % (10 to 19 years). Some people bite and pick more than others and with varying intensity. It is understandably difficult to define the inclusion criteria, which could further skew data and affect accurate measurement. For this book, I will be conservative, and use the lower range (20%) of Ballinger's findings.

I am often asked if more women than men bite their nails. This is difficult to answer. Given societal pressures on women to maintain attractive hands and fingers, I suspect that more men have the habit. My theory may erroneously presuppose, however, that societal pressures are helpful for suppressing the habit. More men than women admittedly call me, but only by a slight margin. This is possibly because men may be less shy about addressing their habit. I believe that women are equally desirous of a solution, but, owing to the very personal and embarrassing nature of the habit, they may be more hesitant to seek help from a stranger. I will address the specific topic of nail biting prevalence between men and women later in the book.

Nail biting also does not appear limited to any particular geography. As far as I can tell, the habit appears in people of all countries and nationalities. I have heard some people remark that they witness the habit more often in the Western nations than in Asian societies. I have found no substantial evidence to verify this opinion. I work more often with Westerners than with Asians or Latin Americans, but this may be explained by the reluctance of Asian or Latin American people to discuss personal matters with outsiders. Incidentally, an interesting, but dated, study of white and black Navy re-

cruits found no significant difference between these groups
of male recruits (Pennington and Mearin, 1980). Both groups
contained habit owners (23%).

All anyone can really say with any authority about nail
biting is that it is highly common and highly stigmatised. It
is boundary and culturally irrelevant, and unrestricted by
demographics. I believe that it is also a highly misunderstood
behavior. Until additional up-to-date studies are conducted,
the reader can simply understand that he or she is not alone
in the world. At the end of 2003, the world's population stood
at approximately 6.4 billion persons. If we conservatively estimate that 20% of this population is currently biting their
nails, you can rest assured that you are in good, if not crowded,
company.

4

HABIT PATTERNS

In my experience with problem nail biting, I have noticed some related behavior patterns that I feel are helpful in further understanding the habit. I would like to share this information with you so that you can understand your own behavior more clearly. Understanding will yield insight, and insight (combined with the technique that I will share later in the book) will allow you to achieve complete freedom from this habit in a very short time.

NAIL BITING AND AGE

I believe that *nail biting is closely related to age.* Nail biting often starts during childhood, at approximately five or six years of age. It can start and stop at just about any age, although the very aged seldom begin biting their nails. I have worked with children, young adults, and middle-aged nailbiters.

The one dominant age pattern that I have recognized is that many more children than adults bite their nails. This assertion is also supported by various clinical studies. For example, in a survey conducted with 78 teachers and 39 schools in South Yorkshire, England, approximately 51% of all school children aged 5-15 years old were nail biters in some degree (Birch 1955). Remember that the estimate for adult nail biting incidence is much lower, at approximately 20% to 30%.

However, I have also worked with middle aged adults who only started to bite their nails following their entry into mid- to late thirties. It is rare though to encounter anyone over the age of 40 who suddenly and spontaneously started biting their nails. It seems that most current habit owners caught the habit when they were young. Although most children naturally quit the habit as they grow older, this book is for those who did not and who continue to suffer from the habit as an adult.

Many people assume that their children or friends will out-grow the habit, and, indeed, this is true. The incidence of nail biting decreases significantly with age, with 14 to 16 being the drop-off point for the vast majority of children (Birch, 1955). However, a significant minority continue to pursue the habit well into adulthood and sometimes for life. I myself did not outgrow it, and many other people have confessed to me that they started as a child and simply continued biting their nails well into adulthood. Many people mention to me that they cannot remember at what age they started. Best guesses indicate that five or six years of age is the most prob-able age.

Although understanding the link between age and nail bit-ing is interesting, the technique I will share is equally effective for any age group except for children under the age of about 15 (more on this later).

MALE AND FEMALE PREVALENCE

I have also observed that *nail biting is somewhat, but not greatly, more prevalent in men than in women.* This is supported by at least one research study with which I am familiar. Reliable, up-to-date data is difficult to locate. Birch (1955) found that for school children, male children under the age of 15 have the advantage (54%) over female children (46%). The difference persists, and research data indicates that it further widens with age.

For example, a separate but somewhat older survey of 1,077 older college students indicated that approximately 29% of the males and 19% of the females surveyed were habitual nail biters (Coleman and McCalley, 1948). These findings indicate to me three things. First, nail biting grows less common as we measure and poll older segments of the general population. Second, that nail biting is generally more prevalent among men. Third, those males tend to outgrow the habit more slowly and at a later age than females. Although more men than women are habitual nail biters, the habit is still quite common in females.

POPULAR BITING TIMES

That nail biting *typically occurs during quiet, inactive times,* is one of the most important patterns that I have witnessed both in myself and in the people that I have helped. Often, nail biting happens when we are in a situation where the mind would like to be exercised.

I will draw a careful distinction here between *why* people bite their nails and *when* they bite their nails. I will address the *why* later in the book. Regarding *when* people bite their nails, I assert that, contrary to popular opinion, primary nail biting does not necessarily happen during periods of high stress or anxiety.

I find that nail biting often takes place while watching TV, riding in a car or at the movies (which was my favourite time to pick). People frequently bite or pick their nails during long and boring meetings or even while on hold on the telephone. Nail biting happens most frequently when the habit owner is alone, bored, or in need of something to do with his or her hands.

Perhaps simply because the hands are engaged, nail biting rarely takes place during sports, physical labour, driving a car, or working at a computer keyboard. Nail biting rarely happens during extremely tense situations. This is curious, given the stereotypical image of a problem nail biter.

This information may be of use or comfort to nail biters who simply wish to be more aware of when and where they bite their nails. The technique that I will give you though, works with anyone, anywhere, and at any time.

Recommendation

If you are a habitual nail biter, I recommend that you begin to keep a personal log or journal indicating the times and conditions under which you engage the habit. You may find the results surprising, and the insight may lead you to faster success when using the technique I am going to describe.

At the minimum, keeping a detailed log of your habit will improve your conscious awareness of the behavior, and reduce the occurrences of unconscious nail biting. Often, nail biting or secondary inspection occurs without realization.

Understanding the conditions under which the habit often appears is useful for drawing our conscious and unconscious minds together. I will share with you a powerful technique for how to do this later in the book.

Just recently, one woman I spoke with was amazed to discover that she only bit her nails after twirling her hair into small curls. Once she understood this behavior link, she ceased both hair twirling and her related nail biting in only a matter of a few days using the technique given below.

5

Am I Causing Damage?

I rarely see nail biting causing any permanent *physical* damage. There will be more about the psychological damage later. However, infections are not uncommon; picking may have broken the skin and open wounds can result from overactive skin pulling. Following a cure, I have occasionally seen some errant re-growth. This is usually easily corrected. Only in very rare cases have I seen nails that are split or that have dropped off.

Our fingernails and toenails are amazingly resilient. They continue to grow even after death. Once the nail-biting habit is cured, no permanent physical damage is evident, even after years of nail biting. In my case, I have no visible scars or indications that I had ceaselessly ravaged my nails and surrounding fingertip skin for many years. Once the habit is broken, roughly forty-five days are required for the nails and skin to re-grow and to become normal. This is even after many, many years of nail biting or picking.

E-mail testimony from a cured subject

> *It is difficult to know how long I bit my nails, since I'm not sure anyone knows when they really start doing it. I certainly have never had nails that went beyond the ends of my fingers! I'm 34 years old, so perhaps 27 or 28 years? It is amazing how easily the nails recover* (Susan, occupation unknown).

More sobering than visible physical damage, however, is possible *physiological* damage. Recently, a link has been drawn between nail biting and lowered IQ in Russian children. Researchers suggest that children in Russia who bite their nails may be ingesting higher than normal levels of lead. As a result of this lead poisoning, their IQs are falling (BBC News, 2003).

Note: if you or your child is a habitual nail biter, I urge you to inspect your home for any traces of older paint that may contain lead. If found, have this paint professionally disposed of to ensure that you and your children do not accidentally ingest any lead.

Continuing, I believe that *the most sinister danger of nail biting is psychological.* Many nail biters that I have seen suffer from lowered self-esteem and an acute sense of embarrassment. This is especially true any time they are discovered publicly pursuing their bad habit. Serious nail biters therefore go to extraordinary lengths to hide their behavior, including clandestine nail picking. Nail biters thus become masters of disguise and concealment when it comes to their habit. Parents should note that criticising or chastising a child nail biter simply drives the child to invent more clever means of hiding the habit. It is counter-productive to criticize any nail biting behavior.

Nail biters frequently suffer from lack of confidence, lowered self-esteem, embarrassment, emotional frustration and occasionally physical pain. They are a misunderstood lot. They feel powerless to stop. They have tried to stop but they keep failing. They feel very alone. This destructive habit has a terrible impact on their self-esteem and confidence.

Consider persons who wish to stop smoking or lose weight. It is much easier said than done. Many people who try to stop smoking cannot endure the withdrawal (chemical or otherwise). They go back to their cigarettes. The first few puffs are absolute bliss. Soon, however, the smoker is consumed by a sense of guilt, disappointment, and discouragement. They shrug their shoulders and admit defeat. This may happen several times in the *life* of a smoker. Imagine though, that it happens several times a *day* in the life of a habitual nail biter. This feeling of helplessness is overwhelming and all-consuming. Indeed, that is how it was for me.

Nail biting creates an insidious and sinister *dark cloud* that hovers pervasively around a person's psyche. After reading this book and curing their habit, many people contact me to say that quitting the habit has removed this cloud. Freedom from the habit releases a great surge of positive energy. This positive energy leads to much higher levels of self-esteem and personal confidence. A strong sense of accomplishment boosts confidence. Often, other unrelated areas of a nail biter's life significantly improve as a result of cured nail biting.

Personal Side Note

Today, I can still remember an incident that occurred in my early childhood. I remember my father towelling me down after a long bath. Taking up one of my hands, he looked troubled and said, "Son, when are you going to stop this horrible habit?" I remember shrugging and responding, "I don't know, Dad. I guess when I grow out of it."

Unfortunately, I never did outgrow it. From that age of six, I habitually and seriously bit my nails until I was in my early 30s. The emotional side of this traumatic habit cannot be understated. I was embarrassed when holding hands with a girl, I had difficulty passing business cards to colleagues and potential clients, and I was continually teased by my friends. I dreaded showing my hands in any situation.

I felt less than whole. I felt powerless to stop. There must be something wrong with a person who would engage in such awful behavior, I thought. I did not know what to do about this horrible and seemingly impossible-to-cure habit. In short, nail biting was destroying my self-esteem and confidence.

I have not bitten my nails since stumbling upon and refining the cure in this book. That was many years ago. Today I continue to attribute higher levels of self confidence to the fact that I was able to break the habit. I feel more in control. I feel more confident when setting higher goals and personal objectives. All of this, I believe, comes from having broken the habit and securing release. Happily, I now feel that there are few challenges in the world that I cannot now at least tackle with a good chance at success. You also will get this feeling after curing your habit.

A Note to Serious Nail Biters

While I consider all cases of nail biting important, there is one class of nail biter to whom I want to send a more specific and serious message. This is the group of nail biters who mention to me that they are a cut above the rest in terms of their habit's voracity. After trying and failing for so long to cure their habit, they remark to me that their problem surely must lie much more deeply than others inside their psyche. Theirs is a more active and sinister case. As a result, there is probably no cure, and no solution. Their case, they say, is frankly hopeless.

To this group of people, I want to say, *don't give up!* From the hundreds of people that I have seen and worked with, I have never seen any person who did more damage to themselves than I did to myself when I was biting my nails. Yes, some cases are more intense than others. However, this simply means that we may have to spend more time on the technique. The desire and motivation to quit should also be correspondingly higher.

However, if pursued with vigour, conviction, and dedication, the cure contained in these pages will work. Do not give this habit any more power than it deserves. It is a simple behavior, and I caution you against giving it omnipotent powers. You can cure yourself. You alone hold the keys to success. Learn the technique and assume responsibility for your cure. Contact me at any time.

6

What Causes Nail Biting?

In this section, I will shed light on possible causes of your problem nail biting. Finding the cause of a problem is often the first step in finding the solution. That being said, though, nail biting is a unique example of a problem whose cure is *not* dependent upon finding the cause of that habit. You will find success regardless of why you bite your nails.

I am frequently asked why is it not necessary to find the cause of the habit in order to cure the habit. The reason is that for many people nail biting was probably caused by some long ago underlying childhood event (possibilities are detailed below). Although that event has long since passed for adult nail biters, the habit has simply persisted as a learned behavior with little continuing relevance to the original catalyst. Since the habit is no longer connected to its roots, curing it often has nothing to do with the reason for its original inception.

This is one reason for why so many people cannot quit the habit. They struggle to find the underlying reason or cause for their habit. This is often an impossible task since those reasons no longer exist. Some nail biters consider their habit so deeply rooted psychologically that a cure is certainly out of the question. They believe they have some mental defect. Again, I say, *hogwash.* You should know that *nail biting is not considered a form of mental illness* in any way, shape or form. It is simply a bad habit. Do not give it any more power than it deserves.

Consider this statement from Ballinger (1970, 446):

> *Members of the normal population and patients in a mental deficiency hospital and a psychiatric hospital were examined for evidence of nail biting. A high prevalence was found in all populations, particularly under the age of 40. It is suggested that nail-biting is* not *an important psychiatric symptom.*

Frankly speaking, there are simply no easy answers to the question, *why do I bite my nails?* There seem to be widely varying opinions regarding the causes of this habit. Type nail biting into any Internet search engine and you will be deluged with information regarding purported causes. This includes stress, boredom, anxiety, self-punishment, grooming, child-hood disorders, and a whole range of other behavior catalysts. The truth is that nail biting may be caused by many factors or by none at all. The reasons for nail biting are as individual and as varied as there are faces in the world. Consider this statement by Pennington (1945, 243):

> *As a result of the interviewing of nearly 7,000 men between the ages of 17 and 37 and as a consequence of the more detailed study of unselected cases of nail biting, it is obvious that the most outstanding finding is diversification of factors responsible for the initiation of this behavior pattern. It follows that a multiple factor interpretation must be used when an overall explanation is sought.*

In laymen terms, nail biting is caused by a wide variety of reasons. There can be multiple causes working in unison, or a single cause is generating the behavior. There is no blanket explanation that can be applied to large or even a small group of problem nail biters.

Pennington continues,

In fact, any specific explanation of nail biting per se, it seems clear, must be based upon an extensive study of each person so addicted. Only in this way can the meaning of the mannerism for the individual personality be determined.

One of the earliest studies on apparent causes of nail biting was conducted in 1929, when family disposition, fatigue, habit formation and fatigue were considered potential causes of problem nail biting (Olson, 1929). In the 1930s, a causal link was investigated between nail biting and sexual activity. Nail biting was postulated as some sort of self-gratification, but the theory ultimately failed to show any scientific basis.

Next, the notion that genetics could somehow be involved in problem nail biting was investigated. An interesting study (Bakwin, 1971) of 203 nail-biting twin children found a surprising basis for the idea that the habit could be genetically related.

Bakwin (1971, 306) states,

The results in twins point to a genetic basis for nail biting. Monozygotic [identical] twins were concordant for the habit about twice as often as dyzygotic [fraternal] twins. Even more striking was the difference when only severe nail biters were studied; the MZ twins were concordant more than four times as often as DZ twins.

A host of other studies throughout the years have also tried to draw a link between nail biting and mental illness or intelligence levels. However, the results of the studies that have been conducted to date indicate that *no one has any real answers*. No one theory, medical diagnosis, or scientific explanation has emerged as a single, identified cause of nail biting. Theories abound, but answers remain elusive. As an informed and intelligent reader, it is up to you to determine the reason for why you bite your nails.

Popular theories are discussed in the following paragraphs. Rest assured, however, that whatever the cause of your nail biting, you will find the solution and the cure in the next chapter.

STRESS AND ANXIETY

This is the most popularly held notion of the reason for problem nail biting among children and adults. At some time in our life, we all have probably nibbled a bit during times of high stress or anxiety. Indeed, this is the classic image of a nail biter. Picture anyone about to make a public speech in front of hundreds and you probably also picture that person biting their nails in a cold sweat.

We are all probably guilty of associating nail biting and stress, and many of us (even among us biters) cling to this stereotypical image. Indeed, we even commonly use the term nail biting as an adjective meaning anxious, stressful or worry full. *The two teams battled to the end in a spectacular, but nail biting finish.* This image persists despite a clear lack of any scientific or medical research to support the association. In my own search, I have yet to find any recognized, medically supported or statistically significant data that indicates that nail biting is caused by stress or anxiety.

It is interesting to explore the anxiety-nail biting link in a bit more detail. First, let us accept that a higher proportion of children than adults bite their nails. To explain this phenomenon, one could attribute high levels of nail biting in children to relatively higher anxiety levels—peer pressure, strict and unforgiving social groups, pressure to achieve school grades, or stifling parental discipline.

Such stressors might explain the high incidence of nail biting in children and young adults. However, is the life of a young child any more stressful than that of a mature adult? And would nail biting be more prevalent within demographics of children who experience abnormal teen stress like broken homes, financial worries, street gangs, etc.? Evidence of this does not exist. Nail biting is prevalent among all children, all demographics.

Further, it seems to me that the older I get, as work and family pressures increase, my own stress levels have increased. If this is so, it would seem to debunk the argument that stress and anxiety are closely linked to nail biting. The incidence of nail biting, instead, *declines with age*. Although my stress levels have increased over the years, I have never again re-lapsed into nail biting. The habit has been permanently and irrevocably erased from my psyche. I will show you how to do the same thing.

Nor have I seen higher rates of nail biting in occupations considered by many to be highly stressful (police, lawyers, corporate executives, etc.). Indeed, persons in less stressful positions bite their nails just as badly. This leads me to be-lieve that stress does not cause nail biting. It may just be an association that was built on preconceived notions and which has survived over time.

If you are a habitual nail-biter, and are spending vast sums on stress reduction therapies for your habit, I suggest that you re-evaluate this approach. Reducing stress is invaluable for avoiding heart disease, but it probably will not affect your nail biting. I heartily recommend any stress reducing activity, but I caution you against placing too much hope in it as a cure for nail biting.

Playing devil's advocate let me propose quite an opposite theory. I assert that the habitual nail biter *first* engages in the behavior and *then* experiences stress *after* he witnesses the damage the habit has caused. Looking back on my own childhood, I do not think that my personal stress levels were any higher than anyone else's. I was a kid like other kids. I doubt that stress caused my habit to materialize. I will say more about this later.

Interestingly enough, the data and profiles that I have collected over the years indicate that most actual nail biting occurs not during times of stress, but *during quiet periods.* People tend to bite their nails while watching TV, attending the movies, or riding in a taxi. If stress or anxiety causes nail biting, why does the behavior occur most often during least stressful activities?

Even I admit, however, that curing the habit improves a person's positive outlook and emotional state. Among the people I have worked with, the cessation of nail biting has a significant calming effect. I liken this to a storm cloud that has suddenly dissipated, leaving bright and sunny skies. The days ahead just seem to be more colourful and free from worry. Once your nail biting is behind you, it is comforting to know that it will never strike again. The anxiety of nail biting is gone.

In summary, it is a common assumption that anxiety causes nail biting. I believe that it is an erroneous assumption. Habitual biters are urged to *not worry* as if quitting the habit was that easy! (Incidentally, the habit is often more difficult to quit than smoking.) I propose to you that the link between nail biting and anxiety may not be as clear cut as perceived. It may actually not exist at all. Alternatively, many people who quit the habit report that they find great pleasure in not having to worry about their nails or habit any longer.

Case Note

Recently, a middle-aged housewife came to me after trying the technique for about three weeks. Her case is shown on the web site, along with *before* and *after* pictures. She told me that her family (in particular, her husband and her nephew) had chided her and told her she was crazy for wasting time on such a cure. She was dedicated though, and diligently stuck with the treatment. Three weeks after our first meeting, I called her to see how she was doing. When she came to visit me at my office, I took the *after* pictures.

Her report to me went something like this:

I really cannot believe that this technique works, but it really does. I am amazed at the progress of my nails, and I really have to say thank you. Although my family doubted me, and my nephew laughed, I stayed true to your technique. I only had to apply the technique a few times, and it worked immediately. I am a little afraid that I might relapse in the future, but I am glad to know that I can always go back to the technique if needed (Sheila, news reporter).

I am not a doctor, nor am I a trained therapist. I am simply a person who bit his nails into a hideous condition for most of his life. I am now habit free and I enjoy wonderful, gorgeous nails. I cannot provide any clinical data to support or refute the apparent causes of nail biting, including anxiety. I can only provide my experience, and the experience of many others who write to me and mention that stress had little to do with their problem habit. I present this material to you *prima facie* for your personal evaluation and applicability to your own situation.

OVERACTIVE GROOMING

That nail biting is caused by some type of evolutionary grooming behavior gone haywire is another theory for why people bite their nails. Although some parents may have serious doubts about their teenage children from time to time, nearly all animals on the planet groom themselves. Grooming, whether done individually or as part of a group, is an integral part of animal and human nature.

We have all seen cats clean themselves, for example, and monkeys grooming each other on television nature programs. People are no different, although our methods of grooming are different from cats and monkeys. We remove our natural oils and replace them with sweet-smelling artificial substitutes. We also cut and clip body hair and nails. Regarding nail biting, then, there is some speculation that nail biting is grooming behavior taken to the extreme.

While this idea may appear ludicrous on the surface, the theory that nail biting is an overactive form of grooming bears further analysis. Remember that I had defined nail biting as a two-step process beginning with the secondary inspection, followed by the primary nail biting.

It is that errant piece of flesh or nail discovered during the inspection [or grooming] that causes the biter to begin engaging his or her nails. What occurs is an intense desire and effort to make the nail or skin smooth and regular.

Many times, I have heard the comment from habitual nail biters that they feel an overwhelming desire or need to *smooth* or prune their fingers to perfection. Irregularities, bumps, edges, grooves, slivers, and hangnails become too much for the biter to bear. They drive him or her mad with preoccupation. The biter simply must clear away the offending irregularity and make the skin and nail smooth and complete.

Personal Side Note

I can still remember what went through my mind every time I went to pick or bite my nails and fingers. First, and often when I was simply bored or thinking of something else, I would inspect. I would inspect in minute detail, turning my fingers this way and that. I would inspect visually, as well as lightly draw a finger over the nail, looking for a bump or an entry point. Often, this behavior was unconscious and I would not even realize it until too late.

After discovery of a flaw, I would get some sort of strange glee in finding a piece of skin or nail that was out of place or that needed pruning. I would arrive then at the jumping off point. Once I found that offending piece of nail or skin, I could not simply let it be there, unattended. I felt an overwhelmingly powerful sense of distraction, a need to clear it away. It became a fixation.

I could not just forget about it. It would stick in my mind as an image, and try as I might, I could not just let it be. I felt certain that if I could only just smooth that one bit, then I would not bite anymore. The area that would be attended to would no longer be out of place.

My thinking was mistaken.

After clearing the offending object, nail biters somehow feel nourished or gratified. They become satiated for the moment. Unfortunately, it is only a temporary fix. The behavior is cruelly cyclical—the more you tear away offending bits, the more disfigured the surrounding skin becomes. This leads to even more offending bits, and the cruel cycle begins anew.

Nail biting is probably some very, very weak form of obsessive-compulsive behavior. We may all experience some weak variant of this condition from time to time. Many of us comb our hair too often, wash our hands too frequently, or vacuum over the same spot countless times.

There are many forms of obsessive-compulsive behavior, and the closest approximation to nail biting might be a habit referred to as *trichotillomania*, or obsessive hair pulling. It would be an interesting exercise to determine if the technique that I outline below would be useful for excessive hair pullers. If you suffer from excessive hair pulling, and have successfully used the technique contained here, please share your experience with us on the public forum. You may help someone else.

SELF-PUNISHMENT

Another theory regarding the cause of excessive nail biting and finger disfigurement is that this form of behavior is some type of self-punishment. As this theory goes, biters feel that they have done something wrong and subconsciously feel the need to hurt or cause themselves pain.

While this may seem far-fetched, when I asked a man who had come to me for help why he thought he bit his nails, he remarked that it was because he felt all biters actually enjoyed the pain in some strange way. Actually, the pleasurable pursuit of pain is more specifically defined as *masochism* and is probably not related to nail biting.

I cannot speak for others, but in my experience I strongly believe that my own nail biting had little to do with self-inflicted pain, punishment, or excessive guilt. I anticipate that the same is true for the vast majority of people who bite their nails—it is simply a bad habit and probably goes no further than that. However, I would be remiss if I did not at least introduce the theory and ask you to examine your behavior and see if there is any relevance. If indeed you feel that there is a connection here, you may wish to seek out professional advice or help.

BOREDOM

A common pattern that I see in *the majority of nail biters* is that *nail biting occurs during moments of boredom, free time, or inactivity.* That is, when nothing in particular is going on, we bite our nails. Nail biting happens most often while watching TV, reading, lying in bed, or lounging at the pool. I frequently bit and picked my nails during taxi rides and at the movies. I believe that this is an important observation. It leads me to believe that boredom has a large role to play in triggering the habit.

I have a regular profession that forces me to fly often to visit clients in neighbouring countries. Looking around on the plane, it is difficult for me to understand how anyone can sit idly in their seat staring at the backrest of the person in front. I need to stay mentally engaged almost all of the time, and I quickly become restless if I have nothing to occupy my mind. Could nail biting be triggered, I wonder, simply by the mind's desire to get up and walk around?

I have presented this theory to many persons who bite their nails, and the amount of support it has received is significant. Many people add their own personal twist; for example, they bite when they are bored but only when there is something pressing on their mind. The theory has credibility. Many nail biters that I have interviewed state that they find it difficult to sit silently without engaging their hands in some way. If their attention is not otherwise engaged, they find it excruciatingly difficult not to pay attention to their nails. Once they start working on their nails, they find it impossible to stop until significant damage is done.

I recognize that there are a good many people in the world who are bored but who do not suffer from the habit. However, from having met and spoken with a large number of nail biters, I can say that many of them simply have trouble occupying themselves when faced with little or nothing to do. If we understand this, we have a good chance at interrupting and modifying the behavior before it results in damaged nails. We can learn to divert our attention and energy to other more productive activities.

Please understand that once you beat the habit, you will not need to fear idle time. Instead, you will learn to embrace periods of relaxation. Curing the habit removes from your mind the need to bite or engage your nails. The habit will not return, no matter how idle your time or your days become. Neither will a new bad habit pop up in its place. I have never seen or heard from anyone any evidence that some strange new habit or tic will arise in place of nail biting once it is cured.

Parent-Child Modelling:

There is support for the theory that nail biting is in part a learned behavior, i.e., children may learn from and imitate the behavior from their parents. Bakwin (1971, 304) states,

The habit is markedly familial. In a large percentage of cases a history of nail biting during childhood by one or both of the parents can be obtained.

I believe that, indeed, some instances of nail biting could be the result of a child imitating its parents. We are the product of our parents in many ways. However, not all cases of nail biting can be explained away so easily. Contradicting myself for the moment, neither of my parents or siblings were habitual nail biters. Neither were my grandparents. If you are a nail biter however, it might be useful for you to investigate whether anyone in your immediate family also has the habit. You might simply have picked it up from them as a child, with no other reasons or sinister causes behind the behavior.

To be safe, I suggest that all parents try to refrain from nail biting in front of their children. I understand that the habit often occurs unconsciously. However, trying to either quit the habit or shielding it from young eyes may help to avoid the habit taking hold in your children while they are young.

7

Cure Your Habit

If you have flipped forward to this chapter without reading and understanding the habit's background as described in the previous six chapters, you have seriously undermined the cure's effectiveness. Many people write to me and indicate that the cure is most effective only when combined with the background reading. You alone are responsible for your own treatment. I strongly recommend going back and completing the reading. Alternatively, if you have diligently completed the reading, I congratulate you. You are about to start your journey to long, gorgeous and healthy nails.

The procedure that I am about to disclose to you requires a high level of personal commitment and dedication. The nail biting habit is very beatable, but only if you are dedicated to following the regimen, completely, honestly, and sincerely.

Biting your nails is your own habit. Nobody else bites your nails (I hope). You are the one person responsible for your own happiness and ultimate success. You started the habit by yourself, and you must now stop the habit by yourself. Together with some help from me, you have the capacity to beat this habit. It is contained within you, but you must learn to find it and exercise it. I will show you how to do the work, but the motivation must come from you. If you are motivated, you will succeed.

The technique is only the tool. By reading this book, you now have access to that tool. Remember, however, that a sharpened chisel is only as powerful as the carpenter who picks it up and uses it to turn blocks of wood into works of art. It is time for you to pick up and use the tool in order to finally, and permanently, rid yourself of nail biting.

The tool is a form of behavior modification referred to as *aversion therapy*. As I mentioned earlier, somewhere deep in your psyche you probably find nail biting somehow gratifying or comforting. If you did not find some satisfaction somewhere deep down, you probably would not bite your nails. Even if you consciously want to stop, your unconscious mind may be sabotaging your efforts. To be effective, a cure must teach both your conscious mind and your deeply buried unconscious that nail biting is no longer gratifying or pleasurable.

In essence, we will take away whatever reward you get from biting your nails. If we do so correctly, the habit will quickly fade and die out a permanent death. You might find it useful to picture the image of a lifeless entity that has had its power source extinguished and which lies motionless on the floor with no hope of recovery.

Read this section several times if you have any doubts or questions. Send me an e-mail if you have any questions or concerns. See also the forum board at http://www.stopyournailbiting.com.

THE SOLUTION

First, find one loose fitting rubber band to wear on your wrist.* It should be loose enough to hang freely, but not so large so that it might fall off. It should also be sturdy enough to withstand stretching to roughly three times its original length.

---

*The author acknowledges and credits the excellent book *Nail Biting: The Beatable Habit*, by Frederick H. Smith, Brigham Young University Press, 1980.

Next, once you are comfortably wearing your rubber band on your wrist …

Draw it out and snap it against the underside of your wrist EACH and EVERY time you either bite your nails or engage in secondary targeting.
BUT DO NOT PRACTICE THIS YET.

As simple as it sounds, this technique is extremely powerful. If you follow the four rules given below, this technique will make nail biting a thing of the past. Please commit the following four rules to memory before starting.

Rule #1: Be Immediate

Immediately upon engaging in either secondary nail inspection or primary nail biting or picking, pull the rubber band back with your opposite hand and let it snap back sharply against the inside of your wrist.

The snap must occur *immediately upon realization that you are inspecting, nail biting, or picking*. We are trying to achieve a very close association in your mind of two things—the nail biting and the minor but sharp pain that you feel when the rubber band snaps against the soft part of the underside of your wrist.

Because the habit is linked closely with the pain, your mind will soon begin to experience a reduction in its desire to bite. We are removing the habit's energy source. We also want to snap immediately, so as to attack the habit at its roots - the secondary inspection. Even if you are not aware of secondary inspection, snap the band as soon as you realize that you are nail biting or primary picking.

Rule #2: Be Forceful

The snap should be hard enough to cause a sharp pain, but not so hard as to cause the skin to break or welt up. If done correctly, the snap will cause a momentary sting, which will travel via the nerve endings up and into your brain. We are conditioning our mind, not torturing our body.

The snap might cause some redness; this is not to worry about. Do not snap hard enough to cause a welt, but do use enough intensity to make you respect the snap. Snap only once for each inspection or nail-biting episode. If you forget to snap on occasion, do not double up next time, but simply be more conscientious in the future with your medicine. You alone hold the keys for your happiness and success.

Rule #3: Be Diligent

It is important that you snap EACH and EVERY time you engage in the habit. That is, snap the band at *each instance* of biting or targeting. Do not let yourself off the hook. This is where your personal commitment is required. Do not become afraid of the band or get lazy. This is the therapy. It is up to you to take your medicine. Be responsible.

Critical Point

We want to be consistent in our therapy. That is, it is important to teach your mind that *every single* instance of either nail biting or targeting will cause a snap—with no exceptions.

If you only snap the band intermittently, then you are significantly (if not completely) negating the power and efficiency of the treatment.

Some readers may be familiar with proven and documented positive and negative reinforcement techniques. Positive reinforcement is most effective when provided only intermittently. Alternatively, negative reinforcement (punishment) is most effective when administered consistently, with assurances that *any* transgression will meet punishment *immediately and consistently.* For an excellent read on the power of positive reinforcement, I suggest *Don't Shoot the Dog* by Karen Pryor (Bantam Books, 1999).

Rule #4: Be Obnoxious

Finally, as you snap the rubber band, hear in your mind a noise so obnoxious that you cringe at the memory of it. By *obnoxious*, I mean frightening, loud, deafening, or whatever it takes to draw your mind's attention to the snap and the pain. We are setting up an alarm in our mind.

I personally use the sound of a fire truck because, for some reason, I find this sound highly annoying and very intrusive. Another friend of mine uses the sound of a metal chair on tiled floor. Ouch! Another person uses the sound of fingernails on a blackboard. Whatever it is, make it *personally offensive* and let it act as a marker to signal that you are now in control of your unconscious thoughts.

This fourth rule will associate the nail biting with both the sound and the band snapping. This will effectively link your conscious and your unconscious and prevent you from biting or preening your nails without being aware of what you are doing. I cannot understate the importance of this step. Hearing the sound in your mind is a very effective technique for drawing your waking mind to what is happening in your subconscious. Hearing the sound as you snap the rubber band links that sound to the pain of the snap. Since the pain occurred as you were targeting or biting, the sound is also now very closely and permanently linked to your habit. This creates a chain of association between the sound, the pain, and the habit. If you perform the technique repeatedly, soon enough you will begin to hear the sound in your mind when you start targeting or biting unconsciously. This technique is a very powerful form of passive protection against unconscious thoughts or nail biting behavior. Your waking mind will quickly be alerted to what is happening in your subconscious.

In its entirety, this technique efficiently and effectively links all of the components together into a very powerful therapeutic approach. By snapping immediately, consistently, and with enough force to cause a sharp but fleeting pain, we have begun to condition the mind that nail biting is no longer a pleasurable or satisfying pursuit. By hearing the sound in our mind, we are also linking this understanding to our subconscious brain so as to guard against engaging the habit without conscious realization.

If you apply the cure consistently and correctly, you will often hear your alarm ringing as you bring your hands up for secondary inspection. Indeed, to this day, I continue to hear the sound in my mind even as I routinely clip or search for dirt under my nails. This is very comforting to me, as I know that I am now and forever guarded against my subconscious. It is like anti-virus software running in the background on your home computer. It is highly effective and convenient passive protection.

When we follow these four rules correctly and with honest commitment, we have a very high probability of success. I have many case examples to support this assertion. Recall also that we have first understood that nail biting is a two-step process. We can now either attack the habit at its root, the inspecting, or we can attack the behavior as it is occurring. Either way, it will be only two or three weeks before you start realizing that you are no longer nail biting.

Note: while you are wearing the band, you do not have to be preoccupied with forcing yourself to quit. The technique does not rely on will power, nor does it matter if you bite your nails during the therapy. If followed correctly, the procedure will result in a natural and almost unnoticed cessation of nail biting.

Although I also address these questions in the FAQs section later in this book, I will pause here and answer two questions that come up repeatedly.

Will I wear the rubber band forever?

No. You may remove it once you are comfortable that you are no longer either inspecting or nail biting/picking. This will take approximately three weeks, but possibly longer or shorter, depending upon your condition. Once you are comfortable in the fact that you are no longer preoccupied with your nails, start to slowly remove the rubber band for one or two hours a day.

Any time you feel as if the habit might reappear, simply wear the band again. In most cases, people remove it completely within two months and never have to wear it again. But you can take comfort in knowing that a rubber band (and treatment) is always within quick reach. Incidentally, remembering the sound in my mind is still comforting to me, even after many years of freedom from this habit. Every now and then, I *practice* hearing the sound in my mind as a good maintenance technique. Occasionaly check the batteries in your fire alarm.

Do I snap even while biting?

Yes, snap the rubber band immediately upon realization that you are inspecting, about to bite, or biting already. The majority of nail biting people do not bite continuously, but pursue the habit in spurts. It is these spurts of behavior that we are focusing on, as well as *each* instance of inspection. **Snap the rubber band immediately as soon as you look down or absent-mindedly draw your fingers up to look for irregularities in the nail or skin.**

Other Tips

The rubber band should be worn 24 hours a day, seven days a week. The band should be worn only when you are prepared to snap it. If you find yourself in a situation where you cannot snap, I suggest that you take off the rubber band until you are again in a position to follow the program.

Again, punishment [aversion therapy] is most effective when performed consistently. Let your mind know that *every* instance of nail biting will *quickly* be met with the sting of the rubber band.

Case Note:

> *One gentleman who was a serious nail biter tried the technique for about three weeks. He had only limited success. I was curious as to why he was not improving. Because the hairs on his arm kept getting painfully entangled in it, he mentioned that he took the rubber band off when he went to bed each night.*
> This was not responsible on his part.
> *I recommended that he wax a small area of his wrist, and continue to wear the band even while sleeping. Upon doing so, he was able to completely quit the habit just two weeks later. He also now understands his wife's leg waxing in a whole new light.*

Further, the choice of which wrist to wear the band on is largely unimportant. I am right handed, so I wore the band on my left wrist. This served two purposes. First, I was able to hide the band under my wristwatch, away from curious eyes. Second, I have more dexterity in my right hand and I can snap more effectively using this hand.

Do not snap the band if you are not biting or targeting. There is no need to practice. Do not be shy about wearing the rubber band in public. If you are queried, simply laugh and mention that it is a reminder of a friend's birthday party or something similar. You will not wear it forever, only for approximately two or three weeks or until you start to notice your progress.

Some people are shy about wearing the band in public. To those folks, I have one question – is not complete and life-long freedom from the habit worth several weeks of band wearing? How about long sleeves for a short spell? It is ok to be creative in your therapy, but be responsible.

Once you have stopped biting, slowly fade the rubber band (remove it). You may remove it slowly, or even completely if you feel in control. If you feel that you are in danger of slipping back into the habit, simply wear the band again and consistently follow the four rules. Eventually, you will remove the band forever.

Finally, it may be useful for habitual nail biters to begin keeping a daily log. Note when and where you engage the habit. This could lend valuable insight into the origins of the habit and provide a better understanding of why the habit took hold in the first place. Understanding the conditions under which the majority of nail biting occurs is helpful for supporting the above therapeutic approach. Some people have found that keeping a log helps them to identify, and therefore avoid, situations where they might start biting their nails again. Once cured though, nail biting will not reappear under any circumstances.

SUMMARY

The technique that I have presented above is effective. For it to be most successful, however, you must follow the four rules sincerely and to the letter. These rules have been developed through trial and error and by identifying factors that support or hinder the cure's effectiveness. If you follow these rules faithfully, I believe that you will be very successful at beating this habit.

You should understand that punishment is an effective treatment in certain circumstances. In general, behaviorists (Baer 1971) have found punishment to be one of the fastest, most effective techniques available for helping people to rid themselves of troublesome behavior. When applied appropriately, punishment can have a dramatic effect on behavior and often yields results that are permanent and irreversible. This is certainly true for nail biting, but only if that punishment is applied consistently. You may object to punishment as a therapeutic approach. However, consider this statement (Baer 1971, 34):

> *Our resistance to the use of punishment is based on moral grounds, not scientific ones. But the moral position that pain is bad and should always be avoided becomes itself immoral when it prevents us from helping persons who have learned behavior that puts them in even greater pain. Unfortunately, many of our public institutions promote just that kind of learning.*

Review:

1. Be consistent. Snap each and every occurrence of either targeting or nail biting. Do not allow yourself to bite without snapping the rubber band. Snap once, and only once, for each occurrence. You will seriously reduce the cure's effectiveness if you snap only intermittently.

2. Be immediate about snapping the rubber band just as you begin to bite your nails. The moment you realize that you are targeting, snap the rubber band. Do not wait 10 or 15 minutes; this will lessen the association of the snap with the habit. If you are targeting or nail biting without realization, do not worry or become stressed. Simply snap the band immediately upon recognition that you are starting into the grooming ritual.

3. Snap the rubber band with enough power and intensity so as to cause a grimace, but not a welt. There may be some slight reddening of the skin area under the wrist, but this will fade in a minute or so. If you find yourself snapping almost continuously (but remember—only one snap for each inspection or biting), keep up the snapping until you are in danger of either drawing blood or causing a skin welt. Typically, enough time goes by between each session of nail biting to allow the wrist area to recover from multiple snaps in one day or even within one hour.

4. Finally, *as you snap, hear in your mind the most excruciating noise* that you can imagine, and at very high volume. Do you remember the sound of somebody's fingernails on a school black board? Then you know what I mean. Hearing this sound will very effectively draw your subconscious attention and prevent you from biting or targeting unconsciously. Keep your anti-virus software maintained and running all the time.

Personal Side Note

At one time in my life, my habit drove me to try anything that would provide even small relief. Thankfully, I noticed that wearing and snapping the rubber band provided a very good reminder and incentive not to bite my nails. I wore the rubber band for 24 hours a day for several months and never took it off. If anyone asked me what I was doing, I simply laughed and ignored their question.

I remember now that I never did fully realize exactly when it was that I stopped biting my nails. It just happened, and I found myself going longer and longer without either biting or picking.

Further, somehow my nails became less of a preoccupation. This is one of the reasons that that the technique is so powerful—it has nothing to do with TRYING to quit. Nor does it have anything to do with will power.

Because I was afraid of the habit reappearing, I continued to wear the rubber band over the next several months despite a complete cessation of the habit. I finally removed it and I have never worn it since. It is still comforting to me though, to know that if I get panicky I can always search around the office and find one. Help is just an arm's length away.

Many people comment to me that simply wearing the rubber band effectively reminds them not to bite. Some people only have to snap for one or two days before the mind wakes up and objects to the treatment by no longer fuelling the habit. Having the band in place provides an excellent and convenient barrier to the habit even without snapping. Once the habit is broken, simply fade the band wearing over the next several weeks.

8

THE PITFALLS OF OTHER METHODS

A simple search on the Internet will reveal that there are a large number of different *cure*s being offered in the market-place. To say that some are dubious would be an understatement. The following material comes from two sources, my own experience, and the experience of hundreds of others that I have spoken to and interacted with.

I have never seen a cure that is as effective, efficient, and simple as the one described here. Nor have I seen any methods or cures that are as well documented with real cases, success stories, and testimonials. Let the facts and data speak for themselves. Let other, less credible solutions fall by the wayside.

The mail I receive on a daily basis is my evidence that nowhere is there a solution that is as perfect as the technique I give in this book. In my mailbox are notes and letters from people who provide verified evidence of their success with this treatment. The support and encouragement I have received from people who have tried the technique prompted me to write this book and share the secret with as many people as possible.

People write to me to express gratitude and to say how lucky they consider themselves for stumbling onto this cure. Many also go into details regarding other methods they tried in the past without success. The following are some of the methods people have told me about. Such methods often fail to deliver on their stated claims. I address each touted remedy according to its prevalence in the marketplace.

BAD-TASTING LOTIONS

I would say that almost 50% of the people who come to me with a nail-biting problem have tried this method. When I consider the number of people in the world who bite their nails, I have to admire the economics involved in this so-called cure. There is some big money here. Unfortunately, too many people fall into this trap simply because they are desperate enough to try anything. I was one of them.

Potential users of this product should know that bad-tasting lotions suffer from four key flaws. One lotion I tried, however, was very effective for keeping my two new stray dogs from chewing on the kitchen cabinets. I am thankful to this company for saving me loads on new cabinets. For habit control though, many nail biters have expressed to me disappointment with this approach.

First, bad tasting lotions do not work well for habitual nail biters who *pick*. This was me. I did not really bite, but I would pick and prune the skin around the nail instead. Obviously then, a bad tasting lotion would not have affected my habit. In my experience, most nail biters also pick. For this reason lotions and creams are only very rarely effective.

Second, bad tasting lotions do not attack the habit at its root. As I revealed in chapter two, nail biting is a two-step process. Bad tasting lotions do nothing to prevent the habitual nail biter from secondary targeting. By default, it is thus not addressing the entire end to end habit.

Third, and perhaps most ironically, bad tasting lotions lose their effectiveness over time. I cannot begin to count the number of people who have remarked to me that they find the lotions curiously tasty, or at least palatable. I have no explanation for this phenomenon, but it is well known that a person's acuity of taste declines with age. The fact that most habitual nail biters are well into their middle age only seems to support my assertion that bad tasting lotions lose their bite over time. (No pun intended.)

At a minimum, many who have used a bad-tasting lotion for a prolonged period remark that they simply grow accustomed to the taste. This is an obvious reduction in efficacy. One woman remarked to me that she had been purchasing this product for several years without any real success. She had no other options and was using the product to make herself feel that she was at least *trying*. This is a very common comment.

Finally, bad tasting lotions and creams wash off. This is probably their biggest flaw, especially for people who are active in sports or who are continually in and out of the water. I was a lifeguard on the coast of Rhode Island for several years, and I can tell you that a bad tasting cream would not have lasted long on my fingers. Long hours spent in boring solitude on the lifeguard chair frequently led to my nail biting.

To all those contemplating purchasing a bad-tasting lotion, I urge you to do a careful and thorough examination of this cure's effectiveness. You may find yourself buying this product forever with no real progress. If so, send me that product's company name so that I can buy the stock and grow rich.

HYPNOSIS

This is probably the second most widely touted remedy for nail biting. While I myself am highly sceptical of hypnosis, there is some evidence that it might be effective for certain disorders or habit management. There seems to be a large pool of people who support hypnotic therapies, and as a non-expert I hesitate to debunk the treatment or alienate millions of supporters of this alternative therapy.

What I will do, though, is share the experiences and comments from other people who have tried this method without success. I once tried a hypnotic tape myself. I fell asleep. As a treatment for insomnia, I have only the highest product endorsement. For nail biting, I suggest that you review your own level of open mindedness.

Regarding hypnosis, one of the first things that I have heard is that many people find their scepticism gets in the way of the treatment. Proponents often remark that if the patient were only more open-minded, the treatment would work. To me, this seems like a roundabout argument. Clear, scientific evidence that hypnosis works would naturally make people more open-minded and the treatment would then gain significant mainstream momentum. Something called an *alternative therapy* does not inspire confidence in my mind.

If you are the type of person who is drawn to serious and well documented clinical data, you may find this treatment method lacks appeal. I have never spoken with one person who has indicated to me that they quit biting their nails after hypnotic therapy.

The second major flaw to the use of hypnosis as a therapy is that it transfers responsibility for the cure to the therapist. The patient's eventual success at overcoming the habit now rests more heavily with the quality or the talents of the hypnotist (or the quality of the product if you have purchased a hypnotic tape).

Nail biting is an extremely personal habit, born from extremely personal reasons. By its nature, the responsibility for quitting the habit must rest with the habit owner. If the hypnotist or hypnotic material is not of sufficient quality or efficacy, the behavior modification results are less assured. Is it not dangerous to rely on the quality of someone else's work for your own cure and well-being?

With regard to the treatment I present in this book, the responsibility for the cure lands squarely on the owner of the habit. This is where I believe it should fall. The car is provided, but the road to success must be travelled by each individual.

Finally, hypnotic tools seem to be perpetual. I have met several folks who tell me that they have been using hypnotic tapes for years. To me, a cure is just that—a cure. It should be final, permanent, and lifelong. Until the benefits of hypnosis are better documented and more widely supported by the scientific and medical community, I retain my scepticism.

BEHAVIOR CHANGE MANAGEMENT

Following creams, lotions, and hypnosis, the next *cure* I have seen touted in the market is what I refer to as *behavior change management*. Here are some examples, and a brief discussion of each supposed therapy.

Incompatible behavior

This technique is very effective for animal training. The trick is to teach the animal to perform a behavior that is incompatible with a second, less desirable behavior. A good example is a dog that jumps on people when guests or visitors arrive. Animal trainers address this problem by teaching the dog to sit (usually with food treats) or to keep four paws on the floor when a guest arrives. This is incompatible with jumping up and helps this annoying dog ownership problem.

For nail biting, the advice is to train or teach yourself incompatible behavior (for example, keep or slap your hands at your sides). There are various versions of this approach (squeezing stress balls, inserting hands into pants pockets). My response to this treatment method is this: if it were this simple, why not just train yourself to stop biting your nails? Many people find that they do not receive the same level of habit gratification from this approach, and as a result often regress quickly back into habitual nail biting. The reason for this is clear. This approach does not teach the mind that nail biting is no longer a satisfying pursuit.

Keep yourself occupied (often used with children)

This is advice to keep yourself or your child engaged in some other type of behavior (e.g., go running) any time the habit rears up. Unfortunately, this advice has several flaws. People, for example, find themselves in down times where they simply relax and contemplate life. It is impossible to stay active 100% of the time. You do not want to go running when you are exhausted and simply want to relax and watch a little TV. In addition, some nail biters engage the habit even when they are very busy or heavily engaged in some activity. You are not going to go running when you have a business deadline to meet. I have found that trying to keeping oneself occupied or distracted, has absolutely no affect on nail biting. The habit persists.

Relaxation techniques or visualization

This form of therapy requires that the patient go off to a quiet place and perform some type of meditation or visualization. The subject meditates and visualizes beautiful, full, well-groomed nails. This technique is designed to negate the nail biting urge and focus the mind on eradicating the habit.

While it is impractical in many ways, this cure has another more serious flaw - the technique is time consuming. Meditation usually takes at least 20 minutes to reach a period of adequate relaxation. Further, I understand that the ability and skill to meditate correctly can take upwards of several years to master.

Brute force

Finally, this method of treatment is one that almost all biters have tried at one time or another. It involves covering up the nails so as to prevent access. In my case, I wrapped a nail or finger in a plastic band-aid for a week or two and hoped that the nail and skin would recover. I pictured myself wrapping each finger one after the next until all ten were recovered and my habit vanquished. It did not work. I actually found myself picking the outside of the band-aid looking for little ways to work under the plastic. Not only was it unsightly, but I would resume the habit immediately after removing the band-aid.

Other people try gloves, but the outcome is the same. The habit has not been treated, only postponed. Such techniques are simply temporary solutions to the problem, not to mention presenting serious intimacy issues for couples. One desperate woman I know had taken to wearing gloves in bed at night. Her husband, although sympathetic, was less than thrilled with this approach.

Nail wraps and polishes

It is not uncommon for female nail biters to apply polish or acrylic nails in a brute force attempt to stop nail biting. I do not recommend this approach. First, this does nothing to treat the underlying habit. Second, polishes and top coats sometimes chip and peel slightly. I have heard that these chips and peelings are similar to bits of skin—they provide additional unnecessary temptation to prune! I do, however, recommend healing or moisturizing lotions. I also suggest frequent trips to the manicurist if your personal economics allows such pampering.

In summary, there is an abundance of advice to nail-biters and varied approaches to treating the problem. Most of it is erroneous and simple old wives' tales. The fact that people continue to come to me seeking help after trying all sorts of different cures (and spending who knows how much money) indicates that these methods leave a lot to be desired. If you are considering or have already tried any form of treatment, please feel free to log onto our site and share your experience with others.

To date, I have not come across any cure that is as effective, efficient, and permanent as the system that I present in this book. It is highly cost effective, simple to perform, fast-acting, ever-present, and has no side effects. It is as close to a perfect cure as I can imagine. A patent for rubber bands is, unfortunately not available. I checked.

9

CASE STORIES

I have many case stories. Here are just four that are also posted on the web site, http://www.stopyournailbiting.com. If you visit the site, you can also see before and after pictures. I will add additional cases to the site as they present themselves.

CASE STORY #1

Sheila contacted me after hearing about the cure from a friend. Her profile was very similar to many habitual nail biters. She had started biting when she was five years old. The habit had never gone away, and had tormented her for many years. She had tried many times to stop and had spent much money on other so-called cures, including a bad tasting lotion.

Sheila was not a biter but a picker. She picked and destroyed the skin around her nails. The bad tasting lotion did not help her habit. She engaged in the habit most often during quiet times, including sitting in the taxi on her way to errands.

She was highly distraught. Her friends and family constantly derided her and often would grab her hands when they saw her engaging in the habit. According to her, "I used to fret badly when I would look down and see my ugly hands."

Although I did not consider her case more serious than others, I did immediately notice that she was suffering. I assured her that we would vanquish this demon quite soon, but I could tell that she was highly sceptical. When asked on a scale of 1 to 10 how badly she wanted to quit, she remarked that her choice would be "off the chart into the teens."

Sheila attended a personal one-on-one nail biting workshop where I present and discuss the method in detail. Following the workshop, she immediately started the technique. I contacted her about three weeks later, and her reply was encouraging.

"For the most part," she told me, "I have stopped biting and picking my fingers, with the exception of the thumbs."

I probed her behavior a bit and reasserted the technique's method. She admitted to having slacked off, but promised that she would resume with more energy as she felt that she was close and did not want any rollback.

About six weeks later, Sheila called me again. This time, she was a different person altogether. She reported that she had quit entirely (even her troublesome thumbs) almost immediately after my follow up call. Apparently, my call had solidified the treatment and given her enough momentum to get over that final hurdle. Her family could not believe the results, and soon after two of Sheila's friends called me for help. Today, Sheila is completely habit free.

"You have no idea how happy I am now that I no longer bite my nails," she told me. "For me, movie times were the worst. I would destroy one or two weeks of growth in less than five minutes! I was truly desperate. Now that I no longer do it, I somehow feel more complete, as if the loop is closed."

CASE STORY #2

Michelle also attended one of my personal workshops. At the time, we took before pictures of her nails, which are posted on the Internet. Her nail biting was mild, but her interest in stopping the habit was high, and therefore encouraging.

Several weeks after the workshop, Michelle came into my office and we took her *after* photos. She mentioned that her husband was visibly impressed by her improvement. At the time, Michelle was still performing the technique, as she still occasionally had the urge to bite. She mentioned, though, that she herself could feel that the habit was close to being eliminated. She promised to continue the technique for another two weeks.

She is now very happy, her nails are improving quickly (you can still see a bit of red around the skin area, but this should disappear very soon), and she is soon to be completely habit free only after three weeks. Never again will this habit bother her.

CASE STORY #3

Just recently, I received an e-mail from Jeffery, who had replied back after I sent him a text message. While compiling a draft of this book, he had contacted me as a result of a friend's referral. Although I was still working on the rough draft, I gave him a copy of the book for free in return for being able to use his case story. Desperate as he was, he readily agreed to the exchange.

On the day I met Jeff, I could tell he was highly frustrated. As a lawyer, he is required to present a confident and assured appearance. But his fingers told a different story. On a scale of mild to heavy nail biting, he definitely would have ranked as a heavy habitual biter.

The technique he was using was a brute force approach. He always had one or two fingers hidden in band-aids. This was unsightly for someone in his profession. As soon as he would remove the band-aid, he would start biting his nails again with even more energy. He was at his wits' end. After giving him the manuscript, I followed up with him several weeks later. This is what he reported:

> *I was able to quickly absorb the material, and right away, I knew that a cure for me was in simple reach. It was so intuitive; I could not believe that I did not think of it myself. There was no problem for me to perform the trick even when meeting with clients. Some people asked me about it, but I shrugged it off with a laugh.*

> *As you suggested, I followed the rules perfectly. I also took your advice and did not try to stop using will power. I simply let the technique take over. Your advice hit the mark in all areas.*

> *Frankly speaking, when you mentioned that this was almost a perfect cure, I silently thought you were giving me bull. I am glad that I came to you, and I hope that you continue to make this technique available to the world's nail biters.*

Jeffery is now completely habit free, and doing very well. He does not wear the band at all.

CASE STORY #4:

After purchasing an early version of this book via the web site, Susan sent me an e-mail. I have reproduced it here *verbatim*, and I believe that her message is encouraging to other biters. She begins by quoting an older message on the forum board extolling the therapy as a *great way out* [a cure].

Knowing a way out is a great way to describe it.... In my particular case, until I went searching earlier this month and discovered your web site, I had never tried to find a way out. Well, other than complete denial! When someone would notice my nails or if my family asked, "Do you STILL bite your nails," one of my more common brush-offs was, "Well, of all the bad habits I could have, I figure this one isn't such a bad one..." Interesting now for me to realize though I acted like I didn't care, how embarrassed I was to have a client see the condition of my nails or to have a co-worker or friend notice and simply not know what to say to a 34-year-old who still bit her nails. I see now those situations truly made me feel like a child. And I believe now that I never tried to fix the problem because I had no idea how to even begin. So, thank you for your help. I truly appreciate it.

A full week now with no nail biting and I don't miss it one little bit. I haven't had to use the technique for two days, but I do remember it as a reminder for the time being. Now the only time I look at my nails is to see if they've grown any more today!

10

FREQUENTLY ASKED QUESTIONS

Do I need to wear the rubber band forever?

No. In all likelihood, you will only have to wear the band for a maximum of one or two months. Less, if you are feeling confident that your nails are less of a preoccupation. Remove it when you are confident that you have stopped biting your nails. Take comfort, though, in knowing that you can always wear it again in the future if needed. Help is immediately available.

On which wrist should I wear the band?

This is personal preference. It does not matter. I am right handed, so I wore the band on my left wrist. I snapped the underside where I knew it would sting effectively. I also wear a watch on my left wrist, which helped to conceal the rubber band. If you wear a watch, please ensure that the watch does not interfere with the snapping.

Should I snap the top part or lower part of the wrist?

This is also up to you, but I recommend the inner part of your wrist closest to your hand. This is where the skin is the thinnest, and there are multiple nerves just under the skin.

If I cannot snap right away, can I wait until after?

No. The snap should be immediate and as soon as you realize you are targeting or biting or picking. If you cannot snap, do not wear the rubber band. Wear it only when prepared to consistently snap.

Does doubling up the snapping achieve faster results?

No, this is not necessary. It may even cause you undue pain, which will make you less willing to snap the next time. This will reduce the treatment's effectiveness. Snap only once for each secondary or primary nail biting episode. Often, the snap alone will provide a good reminder and prompt you to stop biting for the moment. Give the treatment an opportunity to work, and let it takes its natural progression. You will be surprised by the results.

What if I miss a snap or forget to snap?

Simply resume the program. Try harder next time to remember and to snap cleanly. Do not punish yourself for missing a snap. Relax and understand that the technique will work even if you fudge it here and there. However, remember that you alone are responsible for your own cure and happiness.

What if I am not aware of my nail biting?

This is OK. It is natural. Many people have remarked to me that they sometimes do not even realize that they are biting their nails. However, you must snap the band immediately upon realization. By hearing the sound in your mind, you will slowly start to realize that you are biting, picking, or targeting. You will then be in more control of your behavior. This process will happen naturally. Soon the biting and picking will disappear.

Are there any side effects?

No, there are no side effects. Obviously, do not snap the band so hard that you hurt yourself or cause bleeding or welts. Because there are no side effects, this is as close to a perfect cure as I can imagine. Incidentally, there has never been any scientific or medical data to indicate that some other strange malady will appear in the place of a broken habit. Simply put, you do not have to worry about something else popping up.

Will I relapse after removing the band in the future?

No, you will never relapse. For some reason, once the habit is eradicated, it rarely resurfaces. However, should you be one of the very few persons in which it does resurface, you can simply go back to wearing the rubber band for several days.

Case Note

One lady I treated some time back mentioned that she snapped at most only once or twice after trying the technique. Just wearing the rubber band reminded her of the pain of the snap, and she quit biting her nails in about 48 hours. She completely removed the rubber band in four days.

Wearing the rubber band alone is often enough to reinforce the treatment and keep the habit at bay. I have never had anyone call me back and indicate that they simply cannot control the behavior. This statistic is spread over the hundreds of people with whom I have worked.

Can I use it for children?

This is a complex question. I address it below in the children's section. The simple answer is it depends.

Can I use it to cure other bad habits?

This is also a complex question. I have only seen the technique effective for nail biting (both hands and feet) and cheek biting. I would welcome a discussion around whether or not the technique is useful for cigarette smoking, heavy drinking, overeating, etc. I doubt that the technique would be effective in these circumstances due to the chemical interactions that are probably fuelling these behaviors. Please see the chapter on Prudent Caution.

Can I cut my nails after they start to grow?

Absolutely! Once you have kicked the habit, I urge you to redefine your relationship with your nails. Learn to groom them, apply healing lotions, visit a manicurist, etc. This is also part of the healing process. You should learn to become comfortable with your nails, instead of having them negatively preoccupy your mind.

Can I share this trick with friends?

Yes, by all means. Nail biting is an extremely debilitating and frustrating habit. I have seen the look of helplessness on people's faces, and I urge you to give your friends a full and fair opportunity to quit this habit permanently. This means that you must share this material in entirety and as a complete program.

Do not simply tell nail-biting friends to wear a rubber band on their wrist and to snap it when they feel like biting. This is not being fair to them. Now that you know the secret, you have an obligation to give others an equal and fair chance at success. If you are in doubt, please simply refer them to my web site and I will take care of the rest.

11

REGARDING CHILDREN

Parents frequently contact me on behalf of their children. While I would like to say that the technique can also be used for children, I have not seen strong evidence that this is the case. If your child is currently a nail biter, the following material may be of comfort or benefit.

As I mentioned earlier, a person's success with this method is highly correlated with their desire to quit. Children often take a *ho hum* view of nail biting, and rarely give it as much importance as their parents. Most children are not concerned with their habit and believe that they will outgrow it. Statistics indicate that this is true.

The technique involves a small amount of self-applied pain. While adults can see and appreciate the larger picture, children often do not apply the technique consistently and with enough intensity. I would also hesitate to teach children any form of self punishment, particularly one that administers pain. I have had some limited success with young teenagers, but it is really only after the age of 16 or 17 that the approach is viable. Some children are mature for their age, and desperate to stop habitual nail biting (often a boyfriend or girlfriend is involved). In these circumstances, the technique is effective for them. However, please exercise caution when working with young adults.

A Note to Parents

If your child is a habitual nail biter, do not despair. Trust that you cannot or should not attempt to force your child to quit. Your child must decide when it is time to quit. I recommend simply giving your child time and room to grow out of the habit. Most children do. Nail biting is typically not an indicator of any underlying mental illness, trauma or psychological defect. In fact, nail biting among children is of such high prevalence that some experts consider the habit normal. Massler (1950) mentions,

> *From these studies, it must be assumed by reason of its wide prevalence, that nail biting is 'normal' in children from 4 years of age until adolescence, in the sense that 'normal' indicates average ness or the common place.*

Incidentally, you may know that it has been suggested that nail biting in adults could be a leftover behavior stemming from childhood thumb sucking. It may not just be coincidence that thumb sucking and nail biting both dissipate and originate respectively at roughly the same age in children (3 to 5 years of age). Oral thumb sucking gratification pursued as a child is obviously not available to the adult owing to societal demands. It is suggested that nail biting is a socially accepted alternative to thumb sucking. I leave this for your judgment.

In the event that your child does not outgrow nail biting, you now have a very powerful cure at your disposal for when they grow into adulthood. Just be sure to share the secret with the child in entirety and as a system. Or refer them to my web site.

During my research for this book, I have come across the following tips that you may use while you are waiting out the child's maturation process. You may try them in whole or in part. If you find any that are successful, please log onto the site and share, or feel free to expand the list with your own recommendations. I will post all useful tips.

TIPS AND TRICKS FOR WORKING WITH CHILD NAIL BITERS

- Do not nag, punish, or focus on negativity; criticism is not effective.
- Communicate your sincere offer to help and support.
- Help the child to realize when they are biting or picking.
- Do not add to the child's overall level of anxiety with pressure to quit.
- Understand that quitting must be internally generated by the child.
- Seek out support and information from as many sources as possible.
- If you are nail biter, do not bite or pick in front of your children.
- Positively reward child nail biters for well groomed nails.

It may be useful for you to sit down and openly discuss nail biting with your child. Determining the child's own desire to quit is the first step for understanding your child's thinking. A child that sincerely and actively wishes to stop will be very receptive to positive reward and encouragement.

Criticizing a child who is unconcerned with his habit is usually not effective and may serve only to further entrench the behavior.

Finally, if you suspect that your child's nail biting is symptomatic of a deeper more serious condition, seek professional advice or treatment. However, most children simply bite, and then outgrow the habit. As a parent, you can provide your young-adult child with the means to overcome the habit in the future should it become necessary.

12

PRUDENT CAUTION

I am often asked if the technique that I have presented in this book is applicable to other bad habits. Can it be used as defence against smoking, overeating, drugs, nervous disorders, or any other maladies that negatively affect our day-to-day lives?

In working with a significant number of habitual nail biters and interacting with these people via mail, telephone, and e-mail, I have used and seen the technique effective for habits other than nail biting. This includes cheek biting, toenail biting and picking, lip picking, knuckle cracking, and excessive hair or eyebrow pulling. For these types of behaviors, I believe that the treatment is very effective. For other types of habits or more serious conditions, however, I would exercise caution for two reasons.

First, if you are a habitual nail biter who has kicked the habit and wants to apply the technique in other areas, you risk diluting the treatment relative to nail biting. If you snap the rubber band when you want to smoke, then the band loses its effective link to nail biting. If you are as happy as I was to finally quit this habit, then I believe you would do nothing to harm or lower the treatment's power and efficiency. Seek some other magic bullet!

Second, drug use, overeating, smoking, and alcohol abuse all have a chemical or biological component. To my knowledge, nail biting does not have this chemical consideration,

nor is it likely biologically pertinent (assuming that nail biting is not hereditary).

In my opinion, the technique given in this book would not
be applicable for fighting chemical addictions or other deeply
set emotional traumas. I would be remiss if I did not caution
you against using or depending upon this technique for other
behaviors, and I hereby put you on notice that I have done so.

If you are suffering from a malady that is more serious
than simple nail, toe, or cheek biting, I urge you to seek more
qualified treatment. If you have used the technique for hair
pulling or other nervous tics, I would be happy to hear from
you via the web site.

For those persons who wish to do further reading regarding habit control, I recommend the excellent book *Habit
Control in a Day* by N.H. Azrin and R.G. Nunn (Simon and
Schuster, 1977). This book details and provides a compre-
hensive program for controlling a variety of bad habits,
nervous tics, and stuttering.

13

KEEP IN TOUCH

Thank you for purchasing and reading this book. I am confident that if you follow the procedure exactly as I have described, you will vanquish this habit in only a matter of weeks. Some people have suffered from biting their nails for years. They are consistently amazed that the technique works so quickly and efficiently.

Please visit the web site at http://www.stopyournailbiting.com and feel free to post your comments to the Member Board. A lively discussion of why the cure works and its potential application to other strange habits would be beneficial to the many other habitual nail biters in the world.

Share your experience with this technique and with this program of therapy. Often, I receive notes and words of gratitude from people that have found success with this cure approach. These folks go on to say that they now wish they could help other people with this troubling habit. This public forum is a good and efficient way to spread the message that problem nail biting can be cured.

Good Luck!

14

REFERENCE LIST

Baer, D.M. "Let's take another look at punishment." *Psychology Today*, 5 (5), (1971), 32-37.

BBC News. 2003/03/03. "Nail-Biting 'damages IQ'." http://news.bbc.co.uk/go/pr/fr/-/1/hi/health/2798089.stm.

Bakwin, H. "Nail-biting in twins." *Developmental Medicine & Child Neurology*, 1971, *13,* 304-307.

Ballinger, B.R.. "The prevalence of nail-biting in normal and abnormal populations." *British Journal of Psychiatry*, 1970, *117,* 445-446.

Birch, L.B. "The incidence of nail biting among school children." *British Journal of Education Psychology*, 1955, *25,* 123-128.

Coleman, J.C. and J.E. McCalley. "Nail-biting among college students." *Journal of Abnormal and Social Psychology*, 1948, *43,* 517-525.

Daniels, L.K. "Rapid extinction of nail biting by covert sensitization: A case study." *Journal of Behavior Therapy and Experimental Psychiatry*, 1974, *5,* 91-92.

Horan, J.J., A. M. Hoffman, and M. Macri. "Self-control of chronic fingernail biting." *Journal of Behavior Therapy and & Experimental Psychiatry*, 1974, *5,* 307-309.

Lowry, T.P. "Bedwetting and nail biting in military recruits." *Military Medicine*, 1965, *30,* 786-787.

Massler, M., and A.J. Malone. "Nail-biting – A review." *Journal of Pediatrics*, 1950, *36,* 523-531.

Mastellone, M. "Aversion Therapy: A new use for the old rubber band." *Journal of Behavior Therapy and Experimental Psychiatry*, 1974, *5,* 311-312.

Olson, W.C. *The measurement of nervous habits in normal children.* Minneapolis: University of Michigan Press, 1929.

Pennington, L.A. "The incidence of nail-biting among adults." *American Journal of Psychiatry*, 1945, *102,* 241-244.

Pennington, L.A., and R.J. Mearin. "The frequency and significance of a movement mannerism for the military psychiatrist." *American Journal of Psychiatry,* 1944, *100,* 628-632.

Pierce, C.M. "Nail-biting and thumb sucking." In A.M. Freedman and H.I. Kaplan, eds. *The child: His psychological and cultural development.* New York: Atheneum, 1972.

Smith, Frederick H. *Nail Biting: The Beatable Habit.* Brigham Young University Press, 1980.

Smith, M. "Effectiveness of symptomatic treatment of college students." *Psychological Newsletter*, 1957, *8,* 219-231.

ISBN 1412023b4-5